The Sirtfood Diet:

The Amazing Benefits of Activating Your Skinny Gene, Including Recipes!

By

Josh West

Table of Contents

Introduction

I want to thank you for buying the book *The Sirtfood Diet: The Amazing Benefits of Activating Your Skinny Gene, Including Recipes!*

This book contains proven steps and strategies on how to not only follow the Sirtfood diet but to really understand how and why it works.

Here's an inescapable fact: you will want a diet plan that you can not only use to lose weight perhaps. You will want one that you will find so delicious and so easy to follow that it can become a part of your life.

If you do not understand why a particular diet works or know how you can sustain it after the test period, you most likely will abandon all that you have learned. The other frustrating part of most diets is that most people will gain the weight back afterwards because they don't either know how or do not want to continue to maintain the new lifestyle. This diet is different.

It's time for you to become the most amazingly vital, youthful, and in shape person that you can be. We hope that you enjoy this book as we explore the benefits of the Sirtfood diet!

Chapter 1. What are Sirtfoods?

The Sirtfood Diet book was published in January, 2016. Authors of the book, Aidan Goggins and Glen Matten both have impressive credentials for writing and speaking about such an innovative area of health and nutrition.

Aiden is an Irish pharmacologist and Glen is from England. Both are experts in nutritional medicine. They jointly wrote another book a few years earlier as a critique on the supplement industry. Research on Sirtuins stemmed from their work, as a key to healthy weight and longevity.

Sirtuins are a family of proteins that are in living things, and are heavily involved in metabolic processes in the body. Sirtuins, to put it simply, will increase or decrease the way genes are expressed and then will impact what happens in the cells, tissues and organs. Sirtfoods are high in sirtuin, or more accurately, they are high in the *activators* of sirtuins. They make them bloom and come alive.

Amidst the molecular genetic workings of sirtuins, we are especially interested in how these compounds work to trigger fat-burning, to decrease weight, and to increase longevity. As you can see in this description, this is not just about a fad diet, but rather a researched based plan to get at the body's deeper processes related to our weight and our aging which are interrelated. An overweight body will age more quickly. An aging body will not be able to optimize its metabolism and thus the cycle of aging continues.

There is a promise in consuming more Sirtfoods to activate the miraculous Sirtuins. The promise is in the evidence that Sirtfoods can help to increase or decrease these functions of the human body, and along with other healthy lifestyle habits, they will beneficially increase longevity and contribute to weight loss if these Sirtuins are activated.

Research also is being done of possible Sirtuin activator supplements, but supplements for Resveratrol (which will come up later in the book), which contribute to anti-aging as well, have shown to not be effective so the idea of supplements for Sirtuins is unknown. Many natural foods can easily activate Sirtuins, and this is the premise of the book. There are certain foods that are easily accessible to you, and in combinations, they will present the easiest and most natural ways to increase Sirtuin activation in your body, and to help your genes to express health and longevity.

The list of some known Sirtfoods that are the highest in sirtuin compounds are below, in alphabetical order. Those foods with an asterisk have the highest levels, and are the most beneficial of all.

- Apples
- Arugula
- Blackcurrants*
- Buckwheat
- Capers*
- Celery
- Chicory (red)
- Chili pepper
- Citrus fruits
- Cocoa (dark chocolate)*
- Coffee
- Dates (Medjool)
- Extra virgin olive oil
- Fish oil (Omega-3)*
- Green tea*
- Kale*
- Lavage
- Miso soup, and other soy products
- Olives*
- Onions (red)*
- Parsley*
- Red wine
- Strawberries
- Tofu
- Turmeric*
- Walnuts

These foods are found in most grocery stores and in health food shops. They are not necessarily expensive either. A one-time fancy surf and turf dinner at a restaurant would cost much more than a bulk of many of these on a shopping list!

Chapter 2. How do Sirtfoods and the Diet Work?

The basis of the sirtuin diet can be explained in simple terms or in complex ways. It is important to understand how and why it works however, so that you can appreciate the value of what you are doing. It is important to also know why these sirtuin rich foods help to help you maintain fidelity to your diet plan. Otherwise, you may throw something in your meal with less nutrition that would defeat the purpose of planning for one rich in sirtuins. Most importantly, this is not a dietary fad, and as you will see, there is much wisdom contained in how humans have used natural foods even for medicinal purposes, over thousands of years.

To understand how the Sirtfood diet works, and why these particular foods are necessary, we will look at the role they play in the human body.

Sirtuin activity was first researched in yeast, where a mutation caused an extension in the yeast's lifespan. Sirtuins were also shown to slow aging in laboratory mice, fruit flies, and nematodes. As research on Sirtuins proved to transfer to mammals, they were examined for their use in diet and slowing the aging process. The sirtuins in humans are different in the typing but they essentially work in the same ways and reasons.

There are seven "members" that make up the sirtuin family. It is believed that sirtuins play a big role in regulating certain functions of cells including proliferation (reproduction and growth of cells), apoptosis (death of cells). They promote survival and resist stress to increase longevity.

They are also seen to block neurodegeneration (loss or function of the nerve cells in the brain). They conduct their housekeeping functions by cleaning out toxic proteins and supporting the brain's ability to change and adapt to different conditions, or to recuperate (i.e., brain plasticity). As part of this they also help reduce chronic inflammation, and reduce something called oxidative stress. Oxidative stress is when there are too many cell-damaging free radicals circulating in the body, and the body cannot catch up by combating them with anti-oxidants. These factors are related to age-related illness and weight as well, which again, brings us back to a discussion of how they actually work.

You will see labels in Sirtuins that start with "SIR," which represents "Silence Information Regulator" genes. They do exactly that, silence or regulate, as part of their functions. The seven sirtuins that humans work with are: SIRT1, SIRT2, SIRT3, SIRT4, SIRT 5, SIRT6 and SIRT7. Each of these types is responsible for different areas of protecting cells. They work by either stimulating or turning on certain gene expressions, or by reducing and turning off other gene expressions. This essentially means that they can influence genes to do more or less of something, most of which they are already programmed to do.

Through enzyme reactions, each of the SIRT types affect different areas of cells that are responsible for the metabolic processes that help to maintain life. This is also related to what organs and functions they will affect.

For example, the SIRT6 causes an expression of genes in humans that affect skeletal muscle, fat tissue, brain, and heart. SIRT 3 would cause an expression of genes that affect the kidneys, liver, brain and heart.

If we tie these concepts together, you can see that the Sirtuin proteins can change the expression of genes, and in the case of the Sirtfood diet we care about how sirtuins can turn off those genes that are responsible for speeding up aging and for weight management.

The other aspect to this conversation of sirtuins is the function and the power of calorie restriction on the human body. Calorie restriction is simply eating less calories. This, coupled with exercise and reducing stress is usually a combination for weight loss. Calorie restriction has also proven across much research in animals and humans to increase one's lifespan.

We can look further at the role of sirtuins with calorie restriction, and using the SIRT3 protein which has a role in metabolism and aging. Amongst all of the effects of the protein on gene expression, (such as preventing cells from dying, reducing tumors from growing, etc.), we want to understand the effects of SIRT3 on weight for the purpose of this book.

The SIRT3 has high expression in those *metabolically active* tissues as we stated earlier, and its ability to express itself increases with caloric restriction, fasting, and exercise. On the contrary, it will express itself less when the body has a high fat, high calorie-riddled diet.

The last few highlights of sirtuins are their role in regulating telomeres and reducing inflammation which also help with staving off disease and aging.

Telomeres are sequences of proteins at the ends of chromosomes. When cells divide these get shorter. As we age they get shorter, and other stressors to the body also will contribute to this. Maintaining these longer telomeres is the key to slower aging. In addition, proper diet, along with exercise and other variables can lengthen telomeres. SIRT6 is one of the sirtuins that, if activated, can help with DNA damage, inflammation and oxidative stress. SIRT1 also helps with inflammatory response cycles that are related to many age-related diseases.

Calories restriction, as we mentioned earlier, can extend life to some degree.

Since this, as well as fasting, is a stressor, these factors will stimulate the SIRT3 proteins to kick in and protect the body from the stressors and excess free radicals. Again, the telomere length is affected as well.

To sum up, all of this information also shows that, contrary to some people's beliefs that in terms of genetics, such as "it is what it is" or "it is my fate because Uncle Joe has something..." through our own lifestyle choices, and what we are exposed to, we can influence action and changes in our genes. This is quite an empowering thought, and yet another reason why you should be excited to have a science-based diet such as the Sirtfood diet, available to you.

Having laid this all out before you, you should be able to appreciate how and why these miraculous compounds work in your favor, to keep you youthful, healthy, and lean If they are working hard for you, don't you feel that you should do something too? Well, you can, and that is what the rest of this book will do for you.

Chapter 3. Getting Started on Sirtfoods

So, after you have just filled your head with more molecular biology information that you probably needed to since high school or college, let us look at next steps of how to proceed with the Sirtfood diet, and also how to fill your refrigerator.

Starting the Sirtfood diet is very easy. It just takes a bit of preparation. If you do not know what Kale is, or where you would find Green Tea, then you may have a learning curve, albeit very small. There is little in the way of starting the Sirtfood diet.

Since you will be preparing and cooking healthy foods, you may want to do a few things the week you start:

1. Clear your cabinets and refrigerator of foods that are obviously unhealthy and that might tempt you. You also will have a very low calorie intake at the start, and you do not want to be tempted into a quick fix that may set you back. Even though you will have new recipes, you may feel that your old comfort foods are easier at the moment.

2. Go shopping for all of the ingredients that you will need for the week. If you buy what you will need it is more cost effective. Also, once you see the recipes, you will notice that there are many ingredients that overlap. You will get to know your portions as you proceed with the diet but at least you will have what you need and save yourself some trips to the store.

3. Wash, dry, cut and store all of the foods that you need, that way you have them conveniently prepared when you need them. This will make a new diet seem less tedious.

One necessary kitchen tool that you will need aside from the actual foods is a juicer. You will need a juicer as soon as you start the Sirtfood diet. Juicers are everywhere so they are quite easy to find, but the quality ranges greatly however. This is where price, function, and convenience comes into play. You could go to a popular department store, or you can find them online. Once you know what you are going after, you can shop around.

The quality of the juicer will also determine the nutritional quality and sometimes the taste of your juice, which we will explain a bit later. Just know that buying a cheap juicer may seem like a good idea now, but if you decide to upgrade later you will have spent more money, and twice. If you buy a good juicer, think of it like an investment into your health. Many people have spent money for a gym membership that went unused for quadruple the cost of one juicer. A juicer won't go to waste.

So, since not all juicers are alike, let us list a few of the features that you want to look for.

Centrifugal juicers:

Centrifugal juicers do just that, they use centrifugal force to spin the food (most like vegetables like carrots, cucumbers, or kale leaves) at high speeds to the side walls, where there are blades. The food is pushed through a sieve and then you have your juice. You have to drink this rather quickly, as you will lose nutrients the longer it is exposed to air (which it already has done as it was spinning), and it oxidizes, as well as a bit of heat from the friction which creates a loss of nutrients and enzymes. This is the whole reason you are juicing, so this point is quite important. You are also left with a lot of solid but very wet pulp as a byproduct, which also means there was a lot of fibrous parts of the plants that the juicer couldn't handle. This is also a missed opportunity for more nutrients. You will also get a lot of (warmish) foam at the top, which some people do not like. It is quick and it is easy however, and it is usually the cheapest of the juicer types. If you must it is better than not having one at all, but if you can make an investment, you will reap your rewards later.

Masticating juicers:

Masticating juicers also do what they say they are. They masticate or chew the food, albeit more slowly than the other type, by pulling it through gears which extract the juice. The machine pushes the pulp out. You would have less pulp with this machine afterwards. There is also less oxidation, and thus, more nutrients. They also can handle other types of foods (which varies by make and model), but that is something you should consider. You will get some foam with this as well, but not as much. These are more expensive, and again, should be looked at as you would an investment that you would not use and toss away. If you want it to last, and you want to get the most from your juicing and take it seriously, you will want to spend a bit more money and get what you really need.

Twin-gear/triturating juicers:

These geared juicers have gears that grind together with millimeters of space left between, to really tear open foods and grind the plants with only a very dry pulp that is left. These are the most nutrient-efficient juicers on the market. They leave virtually no foam and they are nutrient-dense as they are not disturbing the inner plant cells with oxidation. You usually can tell in the look (color) and taste (richer) than other juices. You can use different attachments to make different foods with most brands as well, so they are versatile. These are the highest pricing of most of the juicers in general, and there are also brand variations as with the others.

Note: If all else fails, in a pinch and with a blender you could get away with a (albeit very poor quality) juice by blending the foods, and using a fine mesh to filter the juice that is left. The only problem is that you would be getting a fraction of the nutrients, and also probably a spike in sugar, as very little fiber will be in the juice to help slow down the natural sugar absorption. Use caution.

Some of the juice recipes call for things that are too soft for most juices, such as if you were to use watermelon. You cannot juice a watermelon, so you should definitely use a blender. A good blender that can work quickly, and has a good strong motor will be a good investment as well.

Citrus Juicers

There are also juicers specifically for citrus fruits. These can range from hand held, col-press juicers, to small electric or automatic cold-press juicers. They too vary in quality and price,

You can do a bit of research on the juicers that you may need. It will help engage your more in the process and journey you are about to take!

Storing Juices

The most nutrition from them immediately, you should drink them right away. If needed you can pre-juice, and put them in glass jelly, Mason jars. The wide mouth variety with the plastic lids is good, airtight and non-corrosive.

You can chill your drinks for the day, by resting them on ice packs in an insulated lunch tote or cooler. In extreme cases, you could juice one to three days of them (it is recommended at the maximum for optimal freshness, although you could push it further out

You may also find something to keep the juice chilled even while you are drinking at home. You can put a jar in the refrigerator just before prepping, and after you juice, pour it into one. You can make it a regular ritual of sorts. Have "your glass" that you get ready every day. If you prefer straws, you can even buy yourself a nice, reusable glass straw. None of these things are necessary for the diet, but any juice just tastes so much better when it is not from plastic.

Here are some other tips to help you get started:

Drink your juices as the earlier meals in the day if it helps you. It is a great way to start your day for three reasons.

- It will give you energy for breakfast and for lunch especially. By not having to digest heavy foods, your body saves time and energy usually spent on moving things around to go through all the laborious motions. You will be guaranteed to feel lighter and more energetic this way. You can always change this pattern after the maintenance phase, but you may find that you want to keep that schedule.

- Having fruits and vegetables before starchy or cooked meals, no matter how healthy the ingredients, is the best way to go for your digestion. Fruits and vegetables digest more rapidly, and the breakdown into the compounds that we can use more readily. Think of it as having your salad before your dinner. It works in the same way. The heavier foods, grains, oils, meats, etc., take more time to digest. If you eat these first, they will slow things down and that is where you have a backup of food needing to be broken down. This is also when you may find yourself with indigestion.

- Juices, especially green juices contain phytochemicals that not only serve as anti-oxidants but they contribute to our energy and mood. You will notice that you feel much differently after drinking a green juice than you would if you had eggs and sausage. You may want to make a food diary and note things such as this!

Be prepared to adjust to having lighter breakfasts for a little while. Most often we fill up with high protein, carbohydrate, and high calorie meals early in the day. We may feel that we did not get enough to eat and that we are not full at first. Oddly as it sounds, we may even miss the action of chewing. Some people need to chew their food to feel like they have had a filling meal. It is something automatic that we do not think of. Some also will miss that crunch such as with toast. Just pay attention to this, and know this is normal, and that it will pass.

Shopping

Now that you have decided on a juicer, let us look at some of the common Sirtfoods that are included in the recipes that were listed earlier, and try to make it easier to prepare. If you can, try to buy fresh, and also organic. Locations may vary, and some things may be purchased bulk. These are some of the top Sirtfoods, and the top-top Super Sirtfoods (with an asterisk*). There are more than are on this list, but these will be the most common ones and the ones that will be mostly used in this book. You can do a Google search and research other Sirtfoods after you get the hang of the plan. Also, see the section on Sirtfood Diet Phases, where you are encouraged to do the plan now and at any time in the future, in addition to staying in the maintenance phase, you can go back to Phases 1 and 2. You can get creative, use these or the different Sirtfoods, and rev up your metabolism again as you would like!

Apples

- Arugula
- Blackcurrants*
- Celery
- Chicory (red)
- Kale*
- Lovage
- Citrus fruits-oranges, grapefruits
- Onions (red)*
- Parsley*
- Strawberries

- Tofu
- Miso soup, and other soy products
- Buckwheat
- Olives*
- Capers* dates (Medjool)
- Extra virgin olive oil
- Walnuts
- Turmeric*
- Cocoa (dark chocolate, 85% or more)*
- Fish oil (Omega-3)*
- Green tea (Matcha preferable)*
- Coffee
- Red wine

In a prior chapter you read about Sirtuins, why they were so important and how they work. These foods above are loaded with them. These foods also have other important qualities for your health such as:

- Vitamins

- Minerals

- Antioxidants, notably catechins, anthocyanins

- Polyphenolic flavonoid compounds such as lutein, zeaxanthin, beta-carotene

- Rutin

- Quercetin

These help work to destroy free radicals, lower oxidative stressors, they are healthy for your heart, brain, and will boost your mood for a plus.

Chapter 4. Sirtfood Diet Phases

The Sirtfood diet has two unique phases designed to do what you have learned Sirtuins will trigger the body to do. It is a fourteen day plan broken up into two phases, where each of the foods or drinks will have their place.

You will start with the lower amount of calories and then gradually increase them. This will jump start your genes and trigger, by way of the Sirtfoods, the Sirtuin proteins to do their job on your "skinny genes."

Phase 1

1,000 Calories

Days 1-3

1. 3 Green Juices

2. 1 cooked Sirtfood meal (SIRT)

Your calories each day of this phase should not go over 1,000. This is your reset   button.

Days 4-7

1. 2 Green Juices

2. 2 Cooked Sirtfood meals

Your calories each day of this phase should not go over 1,500. If followed properly, this phase reports a 7lb. weight loss on average each week.

Phase 2

1,500 Calories

This is a 14-day maintenance plan whereby you do not focus on restricting calories, but you must have at least one green juice. The rest are SIRT meals.

This diet is unlike other diets where it does not end, it truly becomes a part of your lifestyle and could be a permanent way of eating. There would be no restrictions after the traditional diet has ended.

To begin the first phase, simply follow the instructions in the Getting Started on Sirtfoods chapter.

- Purchase your food items based off of the recipes that you think you will like.
- Some of the foods will become staples, so you may always want to keep them around.
- Prepare how you will juice.
- Plan when you will cook, including planning around being away from home or work.

  In the next three Chapters you will get a variety of recipes for:

- Sirtfood Smoothies
- Sirtfood Meals

Having the support of friends and family helps when changing any lifestyle or diet. A green smoothie can spark some strange reactions for someone who has never had one, and who is not on this diet either. A child may make faces at a parent drinking one for breakfast, but if given a taste (without looking), they may grow to love them as well.

The best part about the Sirtfood diet is that anyone can enjoy the juices, smoothies, cooked meals, or desserts. They are not restrictive, and you can eat them and get creative with Sirtfood ingredients for the rest of your long and healthy life.

When you get past Phase 2, you can eat from Sirtfoods as you please. The other great thing about the Sirtfood diet is that you can go back to Phases 1 and 2 at any time. You have the tools and you will have the recipes. You will also will feel more confident about creating your own recipes using a variety of Sirtfoods.

Chapter 5.
Sirtfood Green Juices and Smoothie Recipes

For the first phase, days 1-3, you will drink 3 of the green juices or you can pick from any of the green juices and smoothies in the back of this book (under Phase 2 Recipes).

For days 3-7 you will then have 2 of these a day.

In the maintenance phase, Phase 2, you can have regular Sirtfood meals as long as you have one of these each day.

Matcha juice

Serves: 1

Ingredients

- ½ tsp of Matcha powder (or you can use 1 tea bag strongly pre-steeped in a 1/4 cup of water, and cooled)
- 2 handfuls of kale
- Handful arugula
- 2-3 stalks of celery
- ½ granny smith (green, tart) apple
- 3 sprigs parsley
- ½ lemon, but juiced prior

Instructions:

Juice the vegetables and fruit. Squeeze the lemon in afterwards (do not juice it). Stir in the Matcha green tea powder or the chilled green tea afterwards.

Very Green Juice

Serves 1

Ingredients

- 1 kiwi, peeled, halved
- ½ cup pre-pressed apple juice
- ½ ripe pear, cored
- 1 cup baby spinach leaves (pull off stems if you would like)
- ¼ avocado, pitted and scooped out

Instructions

Simply juice until smooth.

Summer Watermelon Juice

Serves 1

Ingredients

- ½ cucumber, halved
- cups baby kale (can remove stems if you like)
- 2 cups of pre-cut watermelon chunks
- 4 mint leaf

Instructions:

Add all to a blender and blend it very well. Enjoy. You cannot juice watermelon!

Banana berry Smoothie

Serves 1

Ingredients

1 banana

1 cup blackberries

1 cup blueberries

2tbsp. natural yogurt

1 cup milk (or soy/almond or rice milk)

Instructions

Add all to a blender and process until smooth.

Matcha Green Tea Smoothie

Serves 2

Ingredients

1 bananas

2 tsp Matcha green tea powder

1/2 tsp vanilla bean (paste or scraped from a vanilla bean pod)

1½ cups milk

4-5   ice cubes

2tsp honey

Instructions

Add all ingredients except the Matcha to a blender. Blend until smooth. Sprinkle in the Matcha tea powder, stir well or blend a few seconds more (or add cooled green tea).

Green-Berry Smoothie

Serves 2

Ingredients:

1 ripe banana

½ cup blackcurrants (take off stems)

10 baby kale leaves (take off stems)

2 tsp honey

1 cup freshly made green tea (dissolve honey first in tea then chill)

6 ice cubes

Instructions:

Dissolve the honey in the tea before you chill it. Cool first, and then blend all ingredients blender until smooth.

Green Grapefruit Smoothie

Ingredients:

1 grapefruit, peeled and deseeded

6 large kale leaves, destemmed

1 green or red apple, cored and destemmed.

1 carrot

½ cup of water (may use more or less for the texture that you like) **Instructions:**

Place everything into a blender, and blend until smooth. Add water if needed.

Green Apple Smoothie

Ingredients:

1 green apple, cored and destemmed and sliced

6 large kale leaves, destemmed

1 orange, peeled

1 stick of celery

Instructions:

Juice the orange separately in a blender and strain, unless you have a citrus juicer/press.

Juice the celery, kale and apple, mix together and stir, or add to a blender and pulse for a few seconds.

Creamy Green Sunshine Smoothie

Ingredients:

1 avocado, pitted and scooped out

1 banana

5 leaves of kale, destemmed

½ cup of pineapple juice

8 oz. of coconut water

Instructions:

Place the liquids then the fruits and veggies into a blender and blend until smooth.

Chapter 6.
Phase 1 Meal Recipes

In Phase 1, you get to have one meal from this list (or one on the back under Phase 2 recipes). In days 4-7 you get to have two.

Pair these versions of the Sirtfood diet author's dishes with a green juice or smoothie depending on the day or week, and you will be a Sirtfood specialist.

Sesame Miso Chicken

Ingredients:

1skinless cod fillet

½ cup buckwheat

½ red onion, sliced

2stalks celery, sliced

10 green beans

cups kale, roughly chopped

sprigs of parsley

1 garlic clove, finely chopped

1 pinch cayenne or ½ chilli

1 tsp. finely chopped fresh ginger

tsp. sesame seeds

teaspoons of miso

1 tbsp. mirin/ rice wine vinegar

1 tbsp. extra virgin olive oil

1 tbsp. of soy sauce

1 tsp ground turmeric

Instructions:

Coat the cod with a mixture of the miso, mirin and 1 teaspoon of the oil and set aside for 30 minutes up to one hour in the refrigerator.

Heat the oven to 400 F, then bake the cod for 10 minutes.

Sautee the onion and stir-fry in the oil that remains along with the green beans, kale, celery, chili pepper, garlic, ginger. Sautee until the kale is wilted but the beans and celery are tender. Add dashes of water if needed to the pan as you go.

Cook the buckwheat according to the packet instructions with the turmeric for 3 minutes. Add the sesame seeds, parsley and tamari to the stir-fry and serve with the greens and fish.

Tofu and Curry

Serves 4

Ingredients:

8 oz. dried lentils (red preferably)

1 cup boiling water

1 cup frozen edamame (soy) beans

7 oz. (1/2 of most packages) firm tofu, chopped into cubes

2 tomatoes, chopped

1 lime juices

5-6 kale leaves, stalks removed and torn

1 large onion, chopped

4 cloves garlic, peeled and grated

1 large chunk of ginger, grated

1/2 red chili pepper, deseeded (use less if too much)

1/2 tsp ground turmeric

1/4 tsp cayenne pepper

1 tsp paprika

1/2 tsp ground cumin

1 tsp salt

1 tbsp. olive oil

Instructions:

Add the onion, sauté in the oil for few minutes then add the chili, garlic and ginger for a bit longer until wilted but not burned. Add the seasonings, then the lentils and stir. Add in the boiling water and cook for 10 minutes. Simmer for up to 30 minutes longer, so it will be stew-like but not overly mushy. You should check the texture of the lentils half way though.

Add tomato, tofu and edamame, then lime juice and kale. Test for when the kale is tender and then it is ready to serve.

Chicken and Kale with Spicy Salsa

Serves 1

Ingredients:

1 skinless, boneless chicken filet/breast

¼ cup buckwheat

1/4 lemon, juiced

1 tbsp. extra virgin olive oil

1 cup kale, chopped

1/2 red onion, sliced

tsp fresh ginger, chopped

tsp ground turmeric

Salsa:

1 tomato

3 sprigs of parsley, chopped

1 tbsp. chopped capers

1 chili, deseeded and minced (use less if desired) Juice of 1/4 lemon

Instructions:

Chop all ingredients above, just for the salsa, and set aside in a bowl.

Pre-eat the oven to 425 F.

Add a teaspoon of the turmeric, the lemon juice and a little oil to the chicken, cover and set aside for 10 minutes.

In a hot pan, slide the chicken and marinade and cook for 2-3 minutes each side, on high to sear it. Then, slide it all onto a baking-safe dish and for cook for about 20 minutes or until cooked (testing for pinkness).

Lightly steam the kale in a steamer, or on the stovetop with a lid and some water, for about 5 minutes. You want to wilt the kale, not boil or burn it.

Sautee the red onions and ginger, and after 4-5 minutes, add the cooked kale and stir for 1 minute.

Cook the buckwheat, adding in the turmeric (see package or look online if it was bought in bulk, for cooking instructions). Serve the chicken along with the

Smoked Salmon Sirt Salad

Ingredients:

1 cup, or ¼ package (if large) of smoked salmon slices (no cooking needed!)

1 avocado, pitted, sliced, and scooped out

10 walnuts, chopped

5 lovage (or celery leaves), chopped

2 celery stalks, chopped or sliced thinly

½ small red onion, sliced thinly

1 Medjool pitted date, chopped

1 tbsp. capers

1 tbsp. extra virgin olive oil

1/4 of a lemon, juiced

5 sprigs of parsley, chopped

Instructions:

Wash and dry salad makings and vegetables, top with salmon.

Lentil Lovage Salad

Serves 1

Ingredients:

1 cup cooked red lentils (prepare in advance, use warmed or at room temperature)

1avocado, pitted, sliced, and scooped out

2cups baby kale, chopped

2 celery stalks, chopped or sliced thinly

½ small red onion, sliced thinly

1 Medjool pitted date, chopped

¼ cup red currants

1 tsp. turmeric

1 tbsp. extra virgin olive oil

1/4 of a lemon, juiced

5 sprigs of parsley, chopped

Instructions:

Add ingredients and toss together gently. Serve.

Chicken, Kale and Lentil Soup

Serves 2

Ingredients:

5 cups of chicken or vegetable stocks

1 chicken breast, chopped (good use for any leftover chicken form other recipes!

1small red onion

2cups of kale, finely chopped

1 cup of spinach, chopped

1 cup of lentils

1 celery stick, chopped

1 carrot, chopped

1 small chili pepper or a dash of cayenne

A dash of salt

1 tsp. of extra virgin olive oil

Instructions:

Cook the lentils according to the package, but taking them out just a few minutes before they would be done. Set aside.

Add the vegetables to a large pot, sauté in a bit of the oil on medium heat. Stir until the vegetables are softer but not cooked through. Add the chicken (precooked and leftover, plain, skinless chicken), add the lentil you had set aside, and cook for 3-5 minutes more. Add a dash of the salt.

Add the stock, turn down to low, and simmer for 20 minutes. Remove from heat. Serve when cooled.

Spicy Asian Noodle Soup

Serves 2

Ingredients:

1 package buckwheat noodles, prepared as instructed on package

1small red onion

2stalks of celery, washed and chopped

1 chunk of ginger, diced

1 clove of garlic, minced

1 cup of arugula

¼ cup basil leaves, wash, dry and then chop

¼ cup of walnuts

1tsp. of sesame seeds

2tbsp. blackcurrants

½ chili pepper

5 cups of chicken or vegetable stock

Juice of ½ lime

1 tsp. extra virgin olive oil

1 tbsp. of soy sauce

Instructions:

Cook the noodles as instructed and set aside.

In a pan, sauté all of the vegetables, ginger, garlic, chili, and nuts for about 10 minutes on a very low heat. Add the stock, and simmer for another 5 minutes. Cut the noodles (roughly) so that they are in a size small enough to eat in a soup comfortably. Add these to the stock, toss in the sesame seeds, lime juice and remove from heat. Cool and serve.

Chapter 7. Phase 2 Recipes

In this phase, you can have any Sirtfood Meal, as long as you have one Sirtfood juice a day.

Included in this Chapter are recipes to help sustain you in the Maintenance Phase, Phase 2. The other great thing about having these recipes for Phase 2 is that you can use them not just in the maintenance phase, to sustain the weight loss and the changes that you worked so hard to see. You can use them forever, really.

If you are really dedicated, you will be able to experiment with different combinations of Sirtfoods, and create your own combinations and concoctions. Sirtfoods are so natural and you have no restrictions as with some of the other diets, that you could constantly find new ways of preparing them. You will also learn of other foods that contain sirtuins and add these to your repertoire.

Again, you could double some of the recipes and store them, but remember to eat them as soon as you can to save all of those perishable and precious anti-oxidant properties!

Breakfast

Green Omelet

234 calories

Serves 1 • Ready in 10 minutes

2 large eggs, at room temperature

1 shallot, peeled and chopped

Handful arugula

3 sprigs of parsley, chopped

1 tsp extra virgin olive oil

Salt and black pepper

Beat the eggs in a small bowl and set aside. Sauté the shallot for 5 minutes with a bit of the oil, on low-medium heat. Pour the eggs in the pans, stirring the mixture for just a second.

The eggs on a medium heat, and tip the pan just enough to let the loose egg run underneath after about one minute on the burner. Add the greens, herbs, and the seasonings to the top side as it is still soft. TIP: You do not even have to flip it, as you can just cook the egg slowly egg as is well (being careful as to not burn).

TIP: Another option is to put it into an oven to broil for 3-5 minutes (checking to make sure it is only until it is golden but burned).

Berry Oat Breakfast Cobbler

241 calories

Serves 2

2 cups of oats/flakes that are ready without cooking

1 cup of blackcurrants without the stems

1 teaspoon of honey (or ¼ teaspoon of raw sugar)

½ cup of water (add more or less by testing the pan)

1 cup of plain yogurt (or soy or coconut)

Boil the berries, honey and water and then turn it down on low. Put in a glass container in a refrigerator until it is cool and set (about 30 minutes or more)

When ready to eat, scoop the berries on top of the oats and yogurt. Serve immediately.

Pancakes with Apples and Blackcurrants

337 calories

Serves 4

Ingredients:

2 apples, cut into small chunks

2 cups of quick cooking oats

1 cup flour of your choice

1tsp baking powder

2tbsp. raw sugar, coconut sugar, or 2 tbsp. honey that is warm and easy to distribute

2 egg whites

1¼ cups of milk (or soy/rice/coconut)

2tsp extra virgin olive oil

A dash of salt

For the berry topping:

1 cup blackcurrants, washed and stalks removed

3 tbsp. water (may use less)

2 tbsp. sugar (see above for types)

Instructions:

Place the ingredients for the topping in a small pot simmer, stirring frequently for about 10 minutes until it cooks down and the juices are released.

Take the dry ingredients and mix in a bowl. After, add the apples and the milk a bit at a time (you may not use it all), until it is a batter. Stiffly whisk the egg whites and then gently mix them into the pancake batter. Set aside in the refrigerator.

Pour a one quarter of the oil onto a flat pan or flat griddle, and when hot, pour some of the batter into it in a pancake shape. When the pancakes start to have golden brown edges and form air bubbles, they may be ready to be gently flipped.

Test to be sure the bottom can life away from the pan before actually flipping. Repeat for the next three pancakes. Top each pancake with the berries.

Granola- the Sirt way

Serves 1

Ingredients:

1 cup buckwheat puffs

1 cup buckwheat flakes (ready to eat type, but not whole buckwheat that needs to be cooked) ½ cup coconut flakes

½ cup Medjool dates, without pits, chopped into smaller, bite-sized pieces

1 cup of cacao nibs or very dark chocolate chips

1/2 cup walnuts, chopped

1 cup strawberries, chopped and without stems 1 cup plain Greek, or coconut or soy yogurt.

Instructions:

Mix, without yogurt and strawberry toppings.

You can store for up to a week. Store in an airtight container. Add toppings (even different berries or different yogurt.

You can even use the berry toppings as you will learn how to make from other recipes.

More Cooked Meals & Salads

Ginger Prawn Stir-Fry

Serves 1

Ingredients:

6 prawns or shrimp (peeled and deveined)

½ package of buckwheat noodles (called Soba in Asian sections)

5-6 leaves of kale, chopped

1 cup of green beans, chopped

5 g lovage or celery leaves

1 garlic clove, finely chopped

1 bird's eye chili, finely chopped

1tsp fresh ginger, finely chopped

2stalks celery, chopped

½ small red onion, chopped

1cup chicken stock (or vegetable if you prefer)

2tbsp. soy sauce

2 tbsp. extra virgin olive oil

Instructions:

Cook prawns in a bit of the oil and soy sauce until done and set aside (about 10-15 minutes).

Boil the noodles according the instructions (usually 6-8 minutes). Set aside.

Sauté the vegetables, then add the garlic, ginger, red onion, chili in a bit of oil until tender and crunchy, but not mushy. Add the prawns, and noodles, and simmer low about 5-10 minutes past that point.

Chicken with Mole Salad

Ingredients:

1 skinned chicken breast

2 cups spinach, washed, dried and torn in halves

2 celery stalks, chopped or sliced thinly

½ cup arugula

½ small red onion, diced

2 Medjool pitted dates, chopped

1 tbsp. of dark chocolate powder

1 tbsp. extra virgin olive oil

2 tbsp. water

5 sprigs of parsley, chopped

Dash of salt

Instructions:

In a food processor, blend the dates, chocolate powder, oil and water, and salt. Add the chili and process further. Rub this paste onto the chicken breast, and set it aside, in the refrigerator.

Prepare other salad mixings, the vegetables and herbs in a bowl and toss.

Cook the chicken in a dash of oil in a pan, until done, about 10-15 minutes over a medium burner.

When done, let cool and lay over the salad bed and serve.

Strawberry Fields Salad

Ingredients

½ cup cooked buckwheat

1 avocado, pitted, sliced and scooped

1 small tomato, quartered

2 Medjool dates, pitted

5 walnuts, chopped coarsely

20 g red onion

1 tbsp. capers

1 cup arugula

1 cup spinach

3 sprigs parsley, chopped

6 strawberries, sliced

1 tbsp. extra virgin olive oil

½ lemon, juiced

1 tbsp. ground turmeric

Instructions:

Use room temperature buckwheat, or serve warm if preferred. Wash, dry and chop ingredients above, finish with the lemon and olive oil and turmeric as a dressing.

Add the buckwheat then the strawberries to the top of the salad.

Sirtfood Soups

Indian Lentil soup

Serves 2

Ingredients:

2 cups of lentils

1 small red onion, minced

1 stalk of celery, finely chopped

1 carrot, chopped

2 large leaves of kale, chopped finely, or 1 cup of baby kale, chopped

2 sprigs of cilantro, minced

3 sprigs of parsley, minced

¼-1/2 chili pepper, deseeded and minced (use more or less to your taste)

1 tomatoes, chopped into small pieces

1 chunk of ginger, minced

1 clove of garlic, minced

5 cups of chicken or vegetable stock

1 tsp. of turmeric

1 tsp extra virgin olive oil

½ tsp. salt

Instructions:

Cook lentils according to the package, removing from heat about 5 minutes before they would be done.

In a sauce pan, sauté all of the vegetables in the olive oil. Then add the chopped greens last. Then add the ginger, garlic, and chili and turmeric powder.

Add the stock and simmer for 5 minutes. Add the lentils, and salt.

Stir in the pre-cooked lentils and cook longer, on a very low simmer, for 25 more minutes. Remove from the heat and cool.

Cut the avocado, remove the pit, and slice it, then scoop out the slices just before eating.

Top with avocado slice, then serve immediately.

Shrimp & Arugula Soup

Serves 2

Ingredients:

10 medium sized shrimp or 5 large prawns, cleaned, deshelled and deveined

1 small red onion, sliced very thinly

1 cup arugula

1 cup baby kale

2 large celery stalks, sliced very thinly

5 sprigs of parsley, chopped

11 clove of garlic, minced

5 cups of chicken or fish or vegetable stock

1 tbsp. extra virgin olive oil

Dash of Sea Salt

Dash of Pepper

Instructions:

Sauté the vegetables (not the kale or arugula just yet however), in a stock pot, on low heat for about 2 minutes so that they are still tender and still crunchy, but not cooked quite yet. You will need to save the cooking time for the next step. Add the salt and pepper.

Next, clean and chop the shrimp into bite-sized pieces that would be comfortable eating in a soup. Then, add the shrimp to the pot, and sauté for 10 more minutes on medium-low heat. Make sure the shrimp is cooked thoroughly and is not translucent.

When the shrimp seems to be cooked through, add the stock to the pot and cook on medium for about 20 more minutes.

Remove from heat and cool before serving.

Chilled Gazpacho

Serves 2

Ingredients:

2 large, or 6 small tomatoes, chopped

1 avocado, pitted, sliced, and scooped out (wait to do this until instructed)

1 medium cucumber, chopped

1 small red onion, chopped

1 cup of arugula, chopped very finely

½ stalk of celery chopped very finely

1 clove of garlic, minced or pressed

½ chilli or a dash of cayenne pepper

1 tsp. lime juice

Dash of sea salt

Dash of pepper

Instructions:

Add the ingredients to a blender, or a food processor, and pulse gently. You do not want to blend too well, or you will make a liquid, as opposed to a soup. The gazpacho should be chunky. After blending, put into the refrigerator for about 1 hour. You can also let this sit overnight.

Just before eating, slice and scoop out the avocado. Ladle half of the gazpacho into a chilled bowl. Add the slices of avocado and serve immediately.

Snacks

In the Sirtfood Diet these bites below, are referred to as *bites*, not dessert plates! Here is a variation of the Sirtfood authors' take on the *bites*.

Sirtfood Truffle Bites

Makes 15-20

Ingredients:

1 cup walnuts

¾ cup of Medjool dates, pitted

½ cup of dark chocolate broken into pieces; or cocoa nibs

2 heaping tablespoons of cacao powder

½ cup of dried coconut

1 tbsp. ground turmeric

1 tbsp. extra virgin olive oil, or coconut oil (preferred)

1 tsp vanilla extract, or a vanilla pod, scraped

1 dash of cayenne pepper

1 dash sea salt (up to 1/8 teaspoon)

2 tbsp. water if needed

Instructions:

Pulse in a food processor the walnuts and chocolate until finely pulverized. Gently blend solid ingredients next and the vanilla. Make a dough. Make rolled balls out of the dough. Add water a few drops at a time only if I is necessary. Do not use too much water, or you will have to go and add more of the other ingredients to compensate. Refrigerate. Store for up to a week. Take them with you to work or when travelling for a quick pick-me-up as well as to quell a sweet tooth.

Spicy Kale Chips

Ingredients:

1 large head of curly kale, wash, dry and pulled from stem 1 tbsp. extra virgin olive oil

Minced parsley

Squeeze of lemon juice

Cayenne pepper (just a pinch)

Dash of soy sauce

Instructions:

In a large bowl, rip the kale from the stem into palm sized pieces. Sprinkle the minced parsley, olive oil, soy sauce, a squeeze of the lemon juice and a very small pinch of the cayenne powder. Toss with a set if tongs or salad forks, and make sure to coat all of the leaves.

If you have a dehydrator, turn it on to 118 F, spread out the kale on a dehydrator sheet, and leave in there for about 2 hours.

If you are cooking them, place parchment paper on top of a cookie sheet. Lay the bed of kale and separate it a bit to make sure the kale is evenly toasted. Cook for 10-15 minutes maximum at 250F.

Sweet and Savory Guacamole

Ingredients:

2 large avocados, pitted and scooped

2 Medjool dates, pitted and chopped into small pieces

½ cup cherry tomatoes, cut into halves

5 sprigs of parsley, chopped

¼ cup of arugula, chopped

5 sticks of celery, washed, cut into sticks for dipping

Juice from ¼ lime

Dash of sea salt

Instructions:

Mash the avocado in a bowl, sprinkle salt, and squeeze of the lime juice. Fold in the tomatoes, dates, herbs and greens. Scoop with celery sticks, and enjoy!

Thai Nut Mix

Ingredients:

½ cup walnuts

½ cup coconut flakes

½ tsp soy sauce

1 tsp honey

1 pinch of cayenne pepper

1 dash of lime juice

Instructions:

Add the above ingredients to a bowl, toss the nuts to coat, and place on a baking sheet, lined with parchment paper. Cook at 250 F for 15-20 minutes, checking as not to burn, but lightly toasted.

Remove from oven. Cool first before eating.

Berry Yogurt Freeze

Ingredients:

2 cups plain yogurt (Greek, soy or coconut)

½ cup sliced strawberries

½ cup blackberries

1 tsp. honey (warmed) ½ tsp. chocolate powder

Instructions:

Blend all of the above ingredients until creamy in a bowl. Place into two glass or in metal bowls that are freezer-safe, and put into the freezer for 1 hour. Remove and thaw just slightly so that it is soft enough to eat with a spoon. Makes two servings.

Conclusion

Thank you again for buying this book!

I hope this book was able to help you to learn and appreciate more about this amazing diet. The Sirtfood diet is not meant to be a fad, rather it is a way of life.

The next step is to test out all of the recipes, and follow along with each of the phases with the proper foods and drinks. Follow the two planned stages, Phase 1 and Phase 2, and you will be guaranteed to enjoy more energy, vitality, a lighter feeling, and on average, about 7 lbs. lighter on the scale each week.

Thank you and good luck!